STUDIES ON THE DEVELOPMENT OF
BEHAVIOR AND THE NERVOUS SYSTEM

Volume 4

EARLY INFLUENCES

STUDIES ON THE DEVELOPMENT OF
BEHAVIOR AND THE NERVOUS SYSTEM

Volume 4

EARLY INFLUENCES

Edited by
GILBERT GOTTLIEB

Psychology Laboratory
Division of Research
North Carolina Department of Mental Health
Raleigh, North Carolina

ACADEMIC PRESS • New York   San Francisco   London   1978
A Subsidiary of Harcourt Brace Jovanovich, Publishers

ACADEMIC PRESS, INC.
111 Fifth Avenue, New York, New York 10003

United Kingdom Edition published by
ACADEMIC PRESS, INC. (LONDON) LTD.
24/28 Oval Road, London NW1 7DX

LIBRARY OF CONGRESS CATALOG CARD NUMBER: 72–12194

ISBN 0–12–609304–0

PRINTED IN THE UNITED STATES OF AMERICA

CONTENTS

Section 1   DRUGS, RADIATION, HORMONES

Hormonal Influences on Brain and Behavioral Development

J. Mal Whitsett and John G. Vandenbergh

Hormonal Mediation of the Effects of Prenatal Stress on Offspring Behavior

Justin M. Joffe

Section 2   NUTRITION

Introduction

Nutritional Influences on Prenatal Brain Development

S. Zamenhof and E. Van Marthens

Experiential Influences on Brain Anatomy and Brain Chemistry in Rodents

Mark R. Rosenzweig and Edward L. Bennett

Section 4 EPILOGUE

LIST OF CONTRIBUTORS

Numbers in parentheses indicate the pages on which the authors' contributions begin.

EDWARD L. BENNETT (289), Department of Psychology, University of California, Berkeley, and Laboratory of Chemical Biodynamics, Lawrence Berkeley Laboratory, Berkeley, California

GREGORY R. BOCK (249), Department of Otorhinolaryngology and Human Communication, University of Pennsylvania, Philadelphia, Pennsylvania

ROBERT M. BRADLEY (215), Department of Oral Biology, School of Dentistry, University of Michigan, Ann Arbor, Michigan

CONSTANCE J. D'AMATO (35), Department of Pathology, University of Michigan Medical Center, Ann Arbor, Michigan

SAMUEL P. HICKS (35), Department of Pathology, University of Michigan Medical Center, Ann Arbor, Michigan

DONALD E. HUTCHINGS (7), New York State Psychiatric Institute, New York, New York

JUSTIN M. JOFFE (107), Department of Psychology, University of Vermont, Burlington, Vermont

PETER LEATHWOOD (187), Research Department, Nestle Products, Technical Assistance Co. Ltd., Lausanne, Switzerland

CHARLOTTE M. MISTRETTA (215), Department of Oral Biology, School of Dentistry, University of Michigan, Ann Arbor, Michigan

MARK R. ROSENZWEIG (289), Department of Psychology, University of California, Berkeley, and Laboratory of Chemical Biodynamics, Lawrence Berkeley Laboratory, Berkeley, California

JAMES C. SAUNDERS (249), Department of Otorhinolaryngology and Human Communication, University of Pennsylvania, Philadelphia, Pennsylvania

JOHN G. VANDENBERGH* (73), Division of Research, North Carolina Department of Mental Health, Raleigh, North Carolina

E. VAN MARTHENS (149), Mental Retardation Research Center, and Brain Research Institute, U.C.L.A. School of Medicine, Los Angeles, California

J. MAL WHITSETT (73), Department of Zoology, North Carolina State University, Raleigh, North Carolina

S. ZAMENHOF (149), Mental Retardation Research Center and Brain Research Institute, U.C.L.A. School of Medicine, Los Angeles, California

---

* Present address: Department of Zoology, North Carolina State University, Raleigh, North Carolina 27607.

PREFACE

The impetus for the present volume came from the realization that it would be valuable to have under one cover a summary of the various exogenous factors that can affect the early development of behavior and the nervous system. Thus, the prenatal and postnatal effects of drugs, radiation, hormones, nutrition, sensory experience, sensory overload (trauma), and environmental enrichment are discussed in some considerable detail in the chapters to follow. Although the list is not necessarily exhaustive, these are topics about which we know a great deal and they are all matters of considerable everyday importance, as well as scientific relevance. Because of the general interest and public health concern of the topics at hand, we have sought to define technical terms and clarify abstruse issues when they are first introduced and, generally, to have the discussion at a basic enough level so that the material can be digested by readers who are not necessarily well versed in the field.

I am very grateful for the valuable assistance of the eight consulting editors for this volume—their names and institutional affiliations are listed earlier, opposite the title page.

GILBERT GOTTLIEB

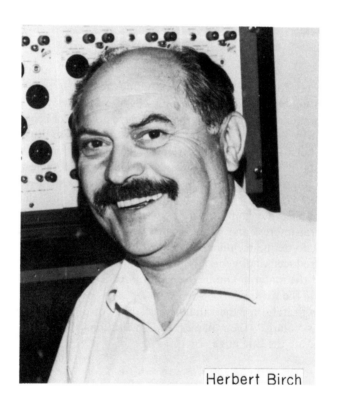

Herbert Birch

DEDICATION TO
HERBERT G. BIRCH (1918-1973)

Herbert G. Birch was a research pediatrician and comparative developmental psychologist of the first order—his professional and research accomplishments span such a variety of fields that they resist easy summary. The very variety of Herbert Birch's research interests makes it especially appropriate to attempt to honor his memory with the volume at hand. His work encompassed the effects of malnutrition, drugs, hormones, trauma, sensory stimulation, and enriched experience, among other factors, on the development of brain and behavior in humans and animals, topics which are the main themes of the present book.

Apparently unable to gain entrance to a medical school in the United States, young Herbert Birch enrolled in the premedical curriculum of the Royal Colleges in Edinburgh, Scotland, in 1937, when he was 19 years old. In 1939, upon the outbreak of the Second World War, he returned to the United States and entered the psychology program at New York University. There he avidly pursued his interests in physiological and comparative psychology, obtaining the B.A. in 1939 and the Ph.D. degree in 1944. (He was to return to the New York University College of Medicine to get his M.D. degree in 1960.)

Herb Birch's early scholarly contacts during graduate school were enviable—he was in touch with the most eminent physiological and comparative psychologists of the generation. As recorded in the preface to his doctoral dissertation, it was while serving as T. C. Schneirla's teaching assistant that Herbert Birch first became interested in "the question of mammalian adaptation." He pursued this interest with chimpanzees at the Yerkes Laboratories of Primate Biology, in Orange Park, Florida, where he conducted his dissertation research with the advice and support of Henry W. Nissen, the assistant director of the laboratories, and Karl S. Lashley, the director of the laboratories. At this late date it is not possible to fathom the administrative arrangement but only to be charmed by its flexibility: Birch was enrolled at N.Y.U. and approved to do his thesis at Orange Park, which was run by Harvard and Yale, without the participation of N.Y.U.

The 1940s marked a particularly fertile intellectual era at Orange Park, one that was to impart a definite and significant direction to both comparative and physiological psychology for years to come. It was indeed a fortunate place for Herb Birch to be at the time. In addition to having contact with Nissen and Lashley, Birch overlapped with postdoctoral research associates Austin H. Riesen, Roger Sperry, and Donald O. Hebb, and could enjoy the frequent visits of such budding luminaries as Frank Beach and William Young. Riesen was in the midst of his now classic dark-rearing experiments with chimpanzees, the results of which were to focus considerable experimental interest on the role of experience in visual perceptual and neural development up to the present day. Sperry was performing his surgical rearrangements of the visual system in amphibians (and, later, nerve transplants in monkeys) which were to continue to serve as the basis for study of the patterning of central–peripheral connections, and the unmodifiability of certain visuomotor coordinations (at least in amphibians) into the 1970s. Hebb was at work on a small monograph which later blossomed into *The Organization of Behavior,* the publication of which, in 1949, inspired the "enriched" early experience approach to problems of perception, learning, and cognition. The publication, in the *Journal of Comparative Psychology* in 1945, of Herbert Birch's thesis on the roles of experience and motivation in the problem-solving of chimpanzees was no small event in the history of that area; it considerably enlarged the perspective of the Gestalt psychologist Wolfgang Köhler, who had inaugurated such research 30 years earlier. This was soon to be followed, in 1945 and 1946, by a three-part article co-authored by George Clark, which opened the area of the hormonal regulation of social behavior in primates: Clark and Birch modified the social-dominance status of male and female chimpanzees upward or downward by hormonal injections.

The intellectual atmosphere of that period at Yerkes is captured very nicely in Austin Riesen's reply to some recent queries.

The Yerkes Laboratories were started jointly in New Haven and in Orange Park, Florida, in 1929, under the title Yale Laboratories of Primate Biology. When Yerkes retired in 1942 the name was changed to Yerkes Laboratories . . ., Lashley assumed the directorship, and Harvard began its joint participation in graduate education there. Yale continued to "keep the books" until 1956 when Emory University took over sponsorship.

As assistant director, Henry W. Nissen, who had sponsored my own dissertation at Yale University, was responsible for my continuing with chimpanzee research and moving to Orange Park a few months after he did in late 1939. He continued to be a strong intellectual guide through all of our deprivation studies, including Herb's. Nissen and I made the first attempts to blindfold a newborn chimpanzee, named Jent, in 1942. We had almost completed the normative observations on an initial group of infants that were nursery-reared. This was to be an experimental animal to be compared with those, but he defeated us by loosening the blindfold in the early morning hours, thereby obtaining unknown amounts of mostly monocular visual experience.

Hebb arrived at Yerkes in 1942. We all had many discussions about Hullian S–R theory, Gestalt theory, and Lashley's healthy and eclectic views by which he found difficulties with both. He had already changed Hebb from a Pavlovian to a man sympathetic to Tolman's and Krech's field-theoretical thinking. Lashley espoused "innatism" and considered our deprivation experiments as not likely to show much of anything.

When Herb arrived in 1942 I was in the Army Air Force High Altitude Training Program, and thus missed much of the period, except for visits of only a few days on widely spaced occasions. Herb Birch and Henry Nissen together persuaded themselves, with some prodding by correspondence from me, to resume the visual deprivation work. They decided that darkroom procedures would be more likely to succeed than using blindfolds.

When I returned to Yerkes in 1946 Hebb was working hard on his *Organization of Behavior*. A monograph, not a hardcover book, was what he had in mind. He, Nissen, and Birch spent many lunch hours discussing factors and brain mechanisms related to earliest behaviors. Lashley was often a participant, but with administrative duties could not always be present.

I am not clear on the details, but I know that Nissen located and recommended Herb for appointment at Yerkes, with Lashley executing the official papers.

Herbert Birch presented his doctoral dissertation to the New York University Graduate School on October 30, 1944. After a further period (1944–1946) at Yerkes as a research associate, in 1947 Birch took an assistant professorship in the Psychology Department of the City College of New York, where he remained until 1955. During the middle and late 1950s, when he once again began pursuing his M.D. degree, Herb Birch evinced his characteristic and marvelously organized "hyperactivity" which allowed him to function effectively while simultaneously holding numerous academic and clinical appointments. For example, during that period, he was an associate clinical professor in the Psychiatry Department of New York Medical College (1954–1960), consulting psychologist to the Department of Physical Medicine and Rehabilitation of the Bird S. Coler Hospital (1953–1960), research associate in the Institute of Physical Medicine and Rehabilitation at the New York University College of Medicine (1955–1956), psychologist-in-charge in the Division of Pediatric Psychology at the Jewish Hospital of Brooklyn (1953–1956), and lecturer in the Psychiatry Department of Columbia University College of Physicians and Surgeons (1956).

With the award of his M.D. degree from the New York University College of Medicine in 1960, Birch began his longtime affiliation with the Department of Pediatrics at the Albert Einstein College of Medicine, first as an associate research professor (1960–1964) and later as a research professor (1964 to his death in 1973). He also held a joint appointment as professor of psychology in the Graduate School of Yeshiva University (1963–1973).

One of the central themes of Birch's research on the psychological development of children concerned the improved communication or intertranslation of perceptual information among the various sense modalities with age and experience. After establishing the normative baselines on the development of intersensory perceptual functioning, he and his colleagues observed that children suffering brain damage or reading disorders or schizophrenia do not manifest the normal degree of intersensory communication and, in some very elementary sense, this lack of competence for intermodal transfer represents their basic perceptual-cognitive deficiency. The point is that the development of increasing competence in synthesizing environmental information from the separate senses is so basic to normal perceptual analysis and appropriate action that a disturbance in such a primary mechanism would inevitably lead to atypical information processing and, thus, to peculiar or "defective" behavior. Birch placed these findings in their full evolutionary context by citing Sherrington's (1941) epic summary of the situation in comparative neurology:

The naive observer . . . would have expected evolution in its course to have supplied us with more various sense organs for ampler perception of the world . . . The policy has rather been to bring by the nervous system the so-called "five" into closer touch one with another. A central clearing-house for sense has grown up . . . Not new senses but better liaison between old senses is what the developing nervous system has in this respect stood for [C. S. Sherrington, *Man on His Nature*, 1941, pp. 278–279].[1]

Speaking of his own developmental work (with A. Lefford) in 1963, Birch had this to say:

Without advancing a recapitulationist argument it is clear that the data of the present study indicate that the phylogenetic evolutionary strategy identified by Sherrington . . . has its counterpart in ontogenetic development. In a sense, the [present] findings are also in accord with the general position advanced by Hebb . . . concerning the slow growth and accretion of per-

---

[1] In light of its seeming general correctness, it is puzzling that Sherrington deleted the "meat" of this extremely important generalization in a subsequent edition of his 1941 work: only the beginning fragment of the quotation can be found in the second edition of *Man on His Nature*, 1951, page 217. Birch was particularly fond of Sherrington's observation and referred to it often in his own writings. It has been a matter of some slight scholarly confusion that Birch always incorrectly cited the 1951 edition as the source for the entire quotation, obviously unaware that Sherrington had changed his mind about the matter in the meantime!

ceptual elements, and suggest one possible mechanism underlying the "sensory spaces" proposed by Piaget . . . as well as the time sequence of their coordination. Most directly they are in accord with the pioneering analysis of the intersensory patterning underlying development advanced by J. M. Baldwin . . . before the turn of the century and with Buhler's . . . view that the phenomenal world of the young child is constructed of well-separated bodies of information deriving from the sensory modalities. . . . Information received by young children through one avenue of sense is not directly transduced to another sensory modality and . . . different age sequences characterize the development of intermodal equivalence among the different senses. In fact, it may perhaps be argued that the emergence of such equivalence *is* development.

Besides authoring more than 150 research articles, commentaries, and chapters, Birch participated in the preparation of six monographs, among which are the following titles: *Intersensory Development in Children* (with A. Lefford), *The Intellectual Profile of Retarded Readers* (with L. Belmont), *Nutrition, Growth and Neurointegrative Development* (with J. Cravioto and E. R. DeLicardie), and *Class and Ethnic Differences in the Responsiveness of Preschool Children to Cognitive Demands* (with M. Hertzig, A. Thomas, and O. A. Mendez). He also co-authored seven books, including *Behavioral Individuality in Early Childhood* (with A. Thomas, S. Chess, and M. E. Hertzig), *Brain Damage in Children* (edited by Birch), *Temperament and Behavior Disorders in Children* (with A. Thomas and S. Chess), and *Disadvantaged Children: Health Nutrition and School Failure* (with J. D. Gussow).

While one is easily overawed by the sheer productivity of Herbert Birch over a 30-year period, it is pertinent to note that he managed to maintain a level of scholarly vigor and clarity that is rarely matched in such a busy and, one imagines, often hectic lifetime. We can only hope that he would have been pleased with our small attempt to honor his memory with the present work.

Section 1

DRUGS, RADIATION, HORMONES

INTRODUCTION

In the first two chapters in this section we are introduced to all manner of "teratogens," foreign substances which, when absorbed or ingested by the pregnant mother during gestation, deform the developing embryo and fetus, even though they may cause the mother little or no obvious harm. Many of these teratogens occur frequently and "normally" in the human environment (X-irradiation, alcohol, prescription and nonprescription medications, vitamins, illegal drugs) and are thus of great public health concern. Depending on when during development (and how much) the embryo or fetus is exposed to the damaging agent or substance, certain predictable structural malformations and/or postnatal behavioral deficits are induced. The principle that is involved is the notion that cells which are actively dividing (proliferating) to form a particular organ at the time of the insult are the ones to suffer most. Different organ systems and parts of the body, brain, and nervous system develop at different times and at different rates, so that is why the specific structural deficits are predictive of the period of gestation (i.e., embryological development) when the insult occurred. These periods are thought of as "critical periods" or "vulnerable periods" of development for obvious reasons. After an organ (or part thereof) has assumed its definitive structural appearance, teratogens no longer cause obvious deformities. Thus, teratogens exert their most obvious and severe damage in the prenatal period, most especially early in the prenatal period in man and other mammals.

As documented by Donald Hutchings in the first chapter and Samuel Hicks and Constance D'Amato in the second chapter, small doses of otherwise teratogenic substances or exposure to various kinds of irradiation, even when they do not cause obvious structural malformations, can have subtle effects on the central nervous system and brain so as to cause borderline or frank mental deficiency and other behavioral problems after birth.

The notions of critical, vulnerable, or "sensitive" periods apply with equal importance to the normal (typical or modal) development of structure, function, and behavior. As shown by Whitsett and Vandenbergh in the third chapter in this section, the appropriate, normally occurring hormones must be available at the right time of organic development if the external sexual organs are to mature properly. Otherwise, genetic males can resemble phenotypic females and vice versa. The "organizing" effect of these hormones on the brain and thus on sexual behavior is not so straightforward, obvious, and temporally delimited, so these authors use the more open term of sensitive period to designate these effects. The brain and central nervous system remain open to hormonal influence well beyond the more limited period of sex-organ formation, and secondary sexual characteristics often remain susceptible to hormonal influence well into adulthood.

These three chapters show us that both normal and abnormal development are equally open to—indeed, are dependent upon—factors extraneous to the genes, cells, tissues, and organs themselves. An awareness of the operation of helpful as well as harmful "extraneous" substances and agents during the prenatal and postnatal periods is necessary to our understanding of both normal and abnormal development.

Since much of the present book shows directly or indirectly that genetic activity is susceptible to "environmental" influence during the course of ontogenetic development, a word needs to be said here about the latest conceptions and experimental findings of ontogenetic developmental analysis, lest the reader who thinks the activity of the genes is immune from such influences become confused or dubious about the obvious implications of the text. Although not widely known or appreciated, it is a fact that genetic activity is turned on and off by hormones (among other things) during the course of development (e.g., O'Malley & Means, 1974; Sara & Lazarus, 1974). Even more striking is the preliminary evidence of Uphouse and Bonner (1975) that DNA activity in the brains of rats is altered by the so-called environmental enrichment procedure described by Dr. Rosenzweig and Dr. Bennett in Section 3. Thus, it is appropriate to designate the new view of the relationship between genes, structure, and function as bidirectional during the course of individual development: genetic activity ⇆ structural maturation ⇆ function.

The implications of this new view for neurobehavioral development have been described at some length elsewhere (Gottlieb, 1976a, 1976b). To the writer's knowledge, this new view of the activity of genes during the course of development has not yet received any mention in a single textbook on behavioral genetics, so there is no wonder that the general reader and student are apt to be unaware of the significant conceptual shift in our thinking about the role of genes in individual development.

References

Gottlieb, G. Conceptions of prenatal development: Behavioral embryology. *Psychological Review*, 1976, **83**, 215–234. (a)

Gottlieb, G. The roles of experience in the development of behavior and the nervous system. In G. Gottlieb (Ed.), *Neural and behavioral specificity*. New York: Academic Press, 1976. Pp. 25–54. (b)

O'Malley, B. W., & Means, A. R. Female steroid hormones and target cell nuclei. *Science*, 1974, **183**, 610–620.

Sara, V. R., & Lazarus, L. Prenatal action of growth hormone on brain and behavior. *Nature (London)*, 1974, **250**, 257–258.

Uphouse, L. L., & Bonner, J. Preliminary evidence for the effects of environmental complexity of hybridization of rat brain RNA to rat unique DNA. *Developmental Psychobiology*, 1975, **8**, 171–178.

BEHAVIORAL TERATOLOGY: EMBRYOPATHIC AND BEHAVIORAL EFFECTS OF DRUGS DURING PREGNANCY

DONALD E. HUTCHINGS

New York State Psychiatric Institute
New York, New York

I. Introduction

Studies of drug consumption among pregnant women both in the United States (Nora, Nora, Sommerville, Hill, & McNamara, 1967; Peckham & King, 1963) and Scotland (Forfar & Nelson, 1973) show that fetal exposure to several medications throughout pregnancy is common. Some preparations, such as vitamins and antacids, are not considered dangerous to the fetus in the recommended dosage but many, including appetite suppressants, tranquilizers, and hypnotics are of questionable safety. Drug abuse, "the self-administration of any drug in a manner that deviates from the approved medical or social patterns within a given culture" (Jaffe, 1975) continues at an all-time high. Alcohol, heroin, amphetamines, and barbiturates head the list of abused agents and illicit methadone now competes with heroin as a drug of choice among addicts (Agar & Stephens, 1975). All of these agents are frequently used in a pattern of polydrug abuse. In New York City alone, conservative estimates indicate that some 3000 infants are born annually whose mothers abused one or more of these drugs during pregnancy (Carr, 1975).

Prenatal drug safety falls within the domain of teratology—the science dealing with the causes, mechanisms, and manifestations of environmentally induced developmental deviations of a structural or functional nature occurring in germ cells, embryos, fetuses, and immature postnatal individuals (J. G. Wilson, 1973). Teratology, however, up until the early 1970s, was concerned almost exclusively with the production of gross structural malformations, with little focus on functional or behavioral manifestations. More recently, however, in the light of clinical observations of infants prenatally exposed to heroin or methadone, but in particular, findings from animal studies in behavioral teratology, it has become increasingly evident that drugs can also produce biochemical or histological damage in the developing central nervous system. These appear to be associated with behavioral effects that include disturbances of arousal (e.g., depression, hyperactivity), specific learning disabilities, impaired motor coordination, and in the case of alcohol, mental retardation. Clinical observations indicate that these effects persist well beyond infancy and the effects produced in animals are typically observed well into adulthood.

The notion that the behavior of infants and children can be affected by drugs taken by the mother during pregnancy is by no means new. Goodfriend, Shey, and Klein (1956) reviewed articles dating back to 1892 which describe opiate withdrawal in the neonate, and Warner and Rosett (1975) cite a medical literature beginning in the early 18th century which warns of increased risk of infant death, "puny" children, and mental deficiency associated with alcohol consumption during pregnancy. The term "behavioral teratology" was introduced by Werboff and his colleagues when they reported a series of studies, beginning in 1961, dealing with the effects on offspring of psychotropic agents administered to pregnant rats. Unlike teratology, however, this field of study has been slow to attract many workers, and has yet to emerge as a well-defined research specialty with a firm theoretical identity. In fact, compared with its "parent" discipline, which has flourished vigorously in the past decade or so, behavioral teratology is just beginning to gather some significant momentum. The reasons for this prolonged gestation are complex, but probably stem in part from historical factors.

Over the centuries, so-called monstrous births have been attributed to a variety of causes: the supernatural, maternal impressions, cohabitation between species, mechanical trauma, developmental arrest, and genetic factors (Barrow, 1971). By the early part of this century, Mendel's work had led to a wide acceptance of a genetic explanation for congenital malformations. Although developmental anomalies had been produced in fish, frog, and chick embryo by irradiation and by mechanical and chemical manipulations, few thought that these observations could be extrapolated to explain human malformations. In fact, it was commonly held that the maternal mammalian organism provided adequate mechanical protection and that the placenta acted as an effective barrier which prevented toxic agents contained in the maternal blood supply from reaching the fetus.

Studies in experimental mammalian teratology began in the early 1930s. Within 10 years, various malformations, previously thought to be genetically caused, had been experimentally induced in the rat by dietary deficiencies (for a review of this early literature, see Warkany, 1965). Further doubt about a strictly genetic explanation of malformations occurred in 1941, when Gregg discovered in humans that rubella contracted in early pregnancy resulted in a syndrome of structural defects that included defects of the brain, heart, and eye. Later workers were to discover postnatal effects that included deafness, dental defects, and mental retardation. A few years later, two chemicals, trypan blue (Gilman, Gilbert, Gilman, & Spence, 1948) and nitrogen mustard (Haskin, 1948) were found to be teratogenic in rats and mice. By the late 1950s, the list of animal teratogens had grown to include, among other substances, aspirin and vitamin A.

In 1961, Warkany and Kalter (1961) reviewed several exogenous factors including viral and bacterial infection, anoxia, and irradiation which had become strongly implicated in the etiology of structural malformations in man. Unable to implicate but a few suspicious drugs, they emphasized the ease with which malformations were experimentally induced by drugs in animals. While aware of the difficulties of extrapolating from animals to man, they nevertheless warned of their potential teratogenic risk.

Warkany's and Kalter's concern presaged the thalidomide disaster which was beginning to unfold as their article was published. This tranquilizer was remarkably nontoxic to the adult in high therapeutic doses but highly toxic to the embryo and ultimately responsible for deforming some 4500 infants in West Germany. Most had severe defects of the extremities, but in addition, many were afflicted with eye, ear, cardiac, intestinal, and urogenital malformations (for review, see Warkany & Kalter, 1964). As the extent of the epidemic became apparent throughout Europe, closer scrutiny indicated that the true proportion of affected infants was nearly double, with about one-third dying soon after birth.

The thalidomide episode caused a long-overdue awakening to the potential danger of careless or indiscriminate use of drugs during pregnancy. Concern over prenatal drug safety was no longer academic. The placenta was finally dethroned as a "barrier" and it became obvious that the embryo could sustain severe nonlethal damage from agents that show little or no toxicity in the adult. These developments in teratology attracted many new workers from diverse specialities, and the field grew rapidly to emerge as a vitally important area of the health sciences.

Historically, behavioral teratology goes back only about 15 years. While much of the early work can be faulted on methodological grounds, one must keep in mind that, at the time, procedural ground rules and organizing theory were lacking. In a series of three studies reported in five articles (Werboff & Dembicki, 1962; Werboff, Gottlieb, Dembicki, & Havlena, 1961a; Werboff, Gottlieb, Havlena, & Word, 1961b; Werboff & Havlena, 1962; Werboff & Kesner, 1963), the antidepressants iproniazid and isocarboxazid, the tranquilizers reserpine, chlorpromazine, and meprobamate, as well as 5-hydroxytryptophan and the benzyl analogue of serotonin, 1-benzyl-2-methyl-4-methoxytryptophan, were administered to pregnant rats at various times during pregnancy. In addition to effects on mortality and morbidity, offspring showed differences in maze learning ability, avoidance conditioning, open-field and inclined-plane activity, and seizure susceptibility. These impairments pointed to behavioral aspects of prenatal drug safety in humans, but stimulated little further work and attracted only a few new workers to the area (for reviews, see Joffe, 1969; Young, 1967).

Several problems may have contributed to the apparent lack of interest. The only thing that appeared to be borrowed from the field of teratology was the name; organizing concepts were not. For example, the behavioral studies indicated that a principle of central importance in teratology, the relationship between developmental stage at the time of treatment and the nature of the effects produced in the offspring, had no relationship to the behavioral changes observed. Moreover, the agents employed were not verified teratogens in the strict sense that they could produce malformations in rat or man. And while the studies assumed that these substances produced biochemical rather than gross morphological alterations in the developing central nervous system, neither biochemical nor histological effects were investigated.

Second, the studies were conceived within the context of intelligent curiosity rather than as experimental tests of specific hypotheses. While such an orientation is both appropriate and understandable as a first step, exploratory studies ultimately must generate testable hypotheses. Each report, however, appeared to end in a kind of cul de sac where it languished, generating few suggestions for new directions.

Finally, these authors voiced genuine concern about the behavioral dimension of prenatal drug safety but never clarified for the clinical practitioner how the animal behavior studied (e.g., maze running, avoidance conditioning, open-field behavior) related to behavioral disorder in infants and children. The studies ostensibly offered an animal model of drug effects on development, but exactly what aspects of human development were incorporated into the animal model remained obscure.

Other studies appeared in the latter part of the 1960s, but most largely failed to replicate the earlier work. The literature progressively became so confused that Joffe (1969), in his critical review, could conclude only that drugs administered prenatally were capable of altering the behavior of the offspring in the absence of gross structural malformations. From an effort that spanned nearly a decade, no systematic relationship between specific kinds of drugs and specific behavioral effects in the offspring emerged.

In the early 1970s the quality of the work improved markedly although quantity remained low. The new investigators were considerably more sophisticated about principles of teratology. They began studying agents that were known to interfere specifically with the histogenesis of the fetal central nervous system; experiments tended to be better controlled and they often described the neuropathology produced by the agents. Some studies even employed behavioral assessment techniques that permitted speculation as to the implications of the behavioral findings for clinical problems in the human population. Some workers suggested that prenatal drug exposure could produce mental retardation; others emphasized the possibility of more subtle effects such as impairment of attention and of motivation. Convincing clinical evidence to support these speculations had yet to appear, however. About this time, retrospective clinical reports began appearing in the literature describing behavioral deviations in infants and children of mothers who had abused alcohol or heroin or who were on methadone maintenance during pregnancy. The effects described ranged from mental retardation (associated with alcohol) to hyperkinesis (associated with heroin and methadone). Most important, however, the behavioral effects persisted well beyond the acute withdrawal reactions which disappeared soon after birth. Thus, the expectations of the early workers in behavioral teratology, expressed some 10 years earlier, were finally being realized.

The present chapter is not an exhaustive review of the behavioral teratology literature. Rather, articles have been selected from the animal literature to elucidate principles of teratology as they apply to functional or behavioral manifestations of prenatally administered drugs. Clinical studies are

reviewed in order to demonstrate the occurrence of similar behavioral
effects in man.

II. Drugs and Prenatal Development: Principles of Teratology and Behavioral Effects

To avoid confusion, the term "teratogenic" will be used here in the narrow
sense to refer specifically to agents which cause gross structural malformation. In the section that follows, it will be shown that some teratogenic
agents, particularly those that interfere with the histological development
of the central nervous system, can produce effects in the absence of gross
structural defects. In the next section, other agents will be discussed that
are not teratogenic in the strict sense of the term but nevertheless produce
behavioral effects, presumably by altering neurochemical and/or hormonal
mechanisms. The proposition will be examined that the following organizing
principles, as outlined by J. G. Wilson (1973), have direct application to the
interpretation of the behavioral effects produced by both teratogenic and
nonteratogenic drugs:

1. The agents act in specific ways (mechanisms) on developing cells and
tissues to initiate sequences of abnormal developmental events (patho-
genesis).

2. The response to toxic agents varies with the developmental stage at the
time of exposure.

3. The effects can include death, malformation, growth retardation, and
functional (behavioral) impairment.

III. Teratogenic Agents

With the exception of a few chemical agents that are of large molecular
size, biotransformed into inactive metabolites by the placenta, or firmly
bound to maternal tissue, most drugs in the maternal circulation readily
cross the placenta and enter the embryonic and fetal milieu. Here, they
activate one or more embryopathic mechanisms which disrupt the inter-
dependent processes of differentiation (i.e., the appearance of new biochemical and structural properties), growth (i.e., the increase in total mass),
and morphogenesis (i.e., the generation of new shape). The embryopathic
result may include death, either directly or secondary to malformation,
malformation that may or may not be compatible with extrauterine life,
growth retardation, and functional alteration that may mediate behavioral
effects. The nature of these effects depends on the specificity and toxicity of
the agent and, most important, on the gestational age or period in development at the time of exposure.

Council of Scientific and Industrial Research, *Annual Technical Report for the Year Ended 31 March, 1954.* Also *Report for Year Ended 31 March, 1953.* C.S.I.R., New Delhi.

Dongerkery, S. R., *A History of the University of Bombay, 1857–1957.* Bombay University Press. 1957.

Dutt, Sunitee, *Prognostic Value of Higher Secondary Examination of Delhi.* C.I.E. Studies in Education and Psychology. Pub. No. 7, Central Institute of Education, Delhi. 1956.

Government of India, Central Institute of Education, *Extracts from the Ordinances & Syllabus for the Master of Education Examination.* Delhi University, 1956.

Extracts from the Ordinances & Syllabus for the Bachelor of Education Examination. Delhi University, 1956.

Government of India, Ministry of Education, *Aims and Objectives of University Education in India.* Pub. No. 157. National Printing Works, Delhi. 1954.

Basic and Social Education, 1956. The Model Press, Ltd.

The Concept of Basic Education. Pub. No. 211, 1956. Kapur Printing Press, Delhi.

Education Quarterly, November 1956. Special Unesco Conference Number. Albion Press.

General Education, Report of the Study Team, 1957. Publication No. 261. Hind Union Press.

Progress of Education in India, 1947–1952. Quinquennial Review. 1953.

A National Plan of Physical Education and Recreation, prepared by the Central Advisory Board of Physical Education and Recreation, Ministry of Education, Government of India, 1956. Publication No. 237. Albion Press.

Indian School of International Studies. *Bulletin of Information,* January 1956–57. Delhi Press.

Report on the Working of the Indian School of International Studies, 3rd October, 1955–2nd October, 1956. University Press, Delhi.

Indian Year Book of International Affairs, 1956, Vol. V, University of Madras. Madras-Diocesan Press. 1956–57.

Kabir, Humayun, *An Indian Looks At American Education.* Eastern Economist Pamphlets, New Delhi. November 1, 1956.

the University of Sydney from the Vice-Chancellor and Principal. Pamphlet. April 1957.

Scarrow, Howard A., *The Higher Public Service of the Commonwealth of Australia.* Duke University Commonwealth-Studies Center, Duke University Press, Durham, N.C. 1957.

Schonell, Professor F. J., *Educational Challenge in a Changing World.* mim. (A.B.C. Talk—24/9/57)

Story, J. D., Vice-Chancellor, *The Committee on Australian Universities,* University of Queensland Gazette, No. 38. September 1957.

The University Amendment Act. University of Queensland Gazette, No. 37. May 1957.

Sydney, University of, Department of Tutorial Classes, *Discussion Groups Syllabus, 1957.* Australasian Medical Publishing Company, Ltd., Sydney.

Forty-Third Annual Report of the Sydney University Joint Committee for Tutorial Classes, 1956. Australasian Medical Publishing Co., Ltd., Sydney.

Department of Tutorial Classes, *Kits, A New Way of Learning Through Group Activities.* Holland & Newton, Printers, Leichhardt. Pamphlet. n.d.

Department of Tutorial Classes, *Some Papers in Adult Education.* Conpress Printing Limited, Sydney. November 1955.

Vice-Chancellor and Principal's Report on the Finances of the University of Sydney. Capital Requirements. April 1957. mim.

CANADA

Banff, School of Advanced Management, *Prospectus for Sixth Annual School of Advanced Management.* February 4 to March 16, 1957.

British Columbia, University of, Department of Extension, *The University Serves Your Community.* 1954. *21st Annual Report, 1956–57.*

Canada, Government of, Reference Papers No. 58. April 16, 1951. *Canadian Universities—Historical.*

Canadian Association of University Teachers, *Brief Submitted to the Royal Commission on Canada's Economic Prospects, January, 1956.* mim.

Canadian Labour Congress and Canadian Association for Adult Education, held at Ottawa, December 1956, *Conference Report, Labour-University Cooperation on Education.*

Dominion Bureau of Statistics, Education Division, *List of Institutions of Higher Education in Canada,* Reference Paper No. 48. Pub. by Authority of the Right Hon. C. D. Howe, Minister of Trade and Commerce. Edmund Cloutier, Ottawa. 1954.

Hall, C. Wayne, and others, *A Century of Teacher Education, 1857–1957.* Institute of Education, McGill University. Pamphlet.

Industrial Foundation on Education, *The Case for Corporate Giving to Higher Education.* Report No. 1. December 15, 1957.

Lower, A. R. M., and others, *Evolving Canadian Federalism,* by A. R. M. Lower, F. R. Scott, J. A. Corry, F. H. Soward and Alexander Brady. Published for the Duke University Commonwealth-Studies Center, Duke University Press, Durham, N. C. 1958.

Manitoba, University of, *President's Report, 1956–57.*

McGill University, *Annual Report for the Year 1955–56.* McGill University and Royal Victoria College, *Statutes Enacted November 28, 1939—Amended to May 31, 1957.* mim.

Meredith, W. C. J., *A Four-Year Law Course On Theoretical and Practical Instruction.* Reprinted from THE CANADIAN BAR REVIEW for October 1953.

Montreal, Ecole Polytechnique, *Modifications au Programme d'Etudes.* n.d.

National Research Council, *Review for 1956.* N.R.C. No. 3976. Ottawa.

Ottawa, University of, *A Catalyst for Science at the University of Ottawa.* Pamphlet prepared by Sponsors' Committee. n.d.

Toronto, University of, *Quarterly for January, 1957.*

Western Ontario, University of, *We Meet the Challenge to Education.* Pamphlet prepared by campaign leaders for fund drive. n.d.

COMMONWEALTH

Bauer, P. T., *Economic Analysis and Policy in Underdeveloped Countries.* Published for the Duke University Commonwealth-Studies Center, Duke University Press, Durham, N. C. 1957.

Jennings, Sir Ivor, *Problems of the New Commonwealth.* Published

for the Duke University Commonwealth-Studies Center, Duke University Press, Durham, N. C. 1958.

Mansergh, Nicholas, and others, *Commonwealth Perspectives* by Nicholas Mansergh, Robert R. Wilson, Joseph J. Spengler, James L. Godfrey, B. U. Ratchford and Brinley Thomas. Published for the Duke University Commonwealth-Studies Center, Duke University Press, Durham, N. C. 1958.

Oliver, Henry M., Jr., *Economic Opinion and Policy in Ceylon.* Published for the Duke University Commonwealth-Studies Center, Duke University Press, Durham, N. C. 1957.

INDIA

Alagappa Chettiar College of Technology, Journal, *Altech.* University Centenary Number. (University of Madras, 1956–57.)

Aligarh Muslim University, Department of Education, *Extension Services for Teachers.* 1956–57.

Bhatia, B. D., *Behavior Problems in Children at Home and School.* Extension Services Pamphlets No. 2, Dept. of Extension Service, Central Institute of Education, Delhi. Kingsway Press. n.d.

Billig, Dr. K. *Research and Building Construction in India.* Bulletin of the Central Building Research Institute, Roorkee. (Council of Scientific and Industrial Research Institute, New Delhi, April 1953, No. 1, Vol. 1.)

Board of Scientific and Industrial Research, *A Review.* Council of Scientific and Industrial Research, New Delhi. 1954.

Bombay, University of, Centenary Souvenir, *University of Bombay, 1857–1957.* Bombay. 1957.

Cadambe, V., *Engineering Research in India.* Council of Scientific and Industrial Research, New Delhi. 1954.

Central Institute of Education, Delhi, *Annual Report, Foundation 1956,* Albion Press. Delhi.

An Experiment in Teacher Education. Publications Division, Ministry of Information and Broadcasting, Central Institute of Education, Government of India. September 1954.

M.Ed. Students, *Short Reports of Studies in Education and Psychology,* Vol. 1, 1952. University Press.

Chandiramani, G. K., *Technological Education in India.* Publication No. 239. National Printing Works, Delhi. 1956.

Education in New India. J. W. Arrowsmith, Ltd., Winterstoke Road, Bristol, England. 1956.

Letters on Discipline. (With a foreword by Jawaharlal Nehru.) Pub. No. 215, Ministry of Education, Government of India. 1956. Albion Press.

Humayun Kabir, *Student Indiscipline.* Ministry of Education, Government of India, 1954. National Printing Works, Delhi.

The Teaching of the Social Sciences in India. Pub. in 1956 by the United Nations Educational, Scientific and Cultural Organization.

Lawrence, H. S. S., *In-Service Teacher Education.* Government of India, Ministry of Education, 1956. Education and Psychology Pub. No. 14, Hind Union Press.

Madras, University of, *History of Higher Education in South India,* Vols. I and II, University of Madras, 1857–1957. Associated Printers (Madras), Private, Ltd., Madras and Bangalore, 1957.

Journal, Section A. Humanities. Centenary Number. Vol. XXVIII, No. 2, January 1957.

Journal, Centenary Number, Vol. 27B, January, 1957.

Annals of Oriental Research, Centenary Number, Vol. XIII, 1957.

Mahajani, G. S., *Our Universities.* Radio talk given on 4/6/56 by the Vice-Chancellor of the University of Delhi.

Mathai, Samuel, *Indian Universities.* Ministry of Education, Government of India, National Printing Works, Delhi. Pub. No. 240. 1956.

Menon, T. K. N. and G. N. Kaul, *Experiments in Teacher Training.* Pamphlet No. 7, Studies in Education and Psychology. Ministry of Education, Government of India, 1954. Government of India Press.

National Council for Rural Higher Education, *Proceedings of the First Meeting.* Pub. No. 254. Agra University Press, Agra.

Sethi, R. R. and V. D. Mahajan, *India Since 1526.* National Printing Works, Delhi. 2nd Ed., 1956.

Seton, Marie, *The Film as an Educational Force in India.* Government of India, Ministry of Education, Culture in Education Series, Pamphlet No. 3, 1956. Coronation Printing Works.

Sidhanta, Sri Mirmalkumar, Vice-Chancellor, Calcutta University, *Address,* January 20, 1957, Calcutta University Centenary Celebration. Calcutta University Press.

Singh, Sohan, *Social Education in India.* Ministry of Education, Government of India, 1956. Pub. No. 253. Messrs. Glasgow Printing Co.

Siqueira, T. N., *The Education of India, History and Problems.* Geoffrey Cumberlege, Oxford University Press, Bombay. 1952.

University of Pennsylvania Bulletin, No. 17, *South Asia Regional Studies.* Vol. LVI, March 15, 1956.

NEW ZEALAND

Adult Education, Council of, Report, *Further Education of Adults.* Wellington, New Zealand. 1947.

Beaglehole, J. C., *The University of New Zealand—An Historical Study.* New Zealand Council for Educational Research. 1937.

Campbell, A. E., *Educating New Zealand.* Centennial Surveys, Department of Internal Affairs, New Zealand, 1941. Wellington.

Culliford, Dr. S. G., Editor, *The Middle District, No. 1.* October 1957. Bulletin.

Currie, G. A., *A Federation of Universities in New Zealand.* Memorandum by the Vice-Chancellor to the Senate, August 10, 1954. *Financing Universities, With Special Reference to Great Britain, Australia and New Zealand.* Mimeographed copy of address given to Officers of the Treasury in 1956 by the Vice-Chancellor of the University of New Zealand.

Report to the Senate on University Entrance, July 19, 1957.

New Zealand, Official Year-Book, 1956, *Education, Section 6.* (An extract) Compiled by the Department of Statistics. R. E. Owen, Government Printer, Wellington, New Zealand. 1957.

New Zealand Department of Education, *Teaching as a Career.* R. E. Owen, Government Printer, Wellington, New Zealand. 1957.

Smith, Sir David, *The External Examiner, The Degree in Agriculture, The University and the Post-Primary Schools, University Education and Specialization.* An address to the Senate of the the University of New Zealand at its meeting at Canterbury Agricultural College, August 23, 1955, by the Hon. Sir David Smith, Chancellor of the University. Publisher not given.

Williams, J., Principal of Victoria University College, *Report of*

Principal on Visits to United Kingdom, United States of America and Canada. mim. April 9, 1956.

PAKISTAN

Government of Pakistan Planning Board, *The First Five Year Plan 1955–60.* Education Training (Draft). May 1956.

UNITED KINGDOM

Armytage, W. H. G., *Civic Universities.* Ernest Benn, Ltd., London, England. 1955.

Ashby, Sir Eric, *Technology and the Academics.* Macmillan & Co., Ltd., London. 1958.

Association of Universities of the British Commonwealth, *United Kingdom Postgraduate Awards, 1955–56,* November 1955. Printed in Great Britain by R&R Clark, Ltd., Edinburgh.
Yearbook of the Universities of the Commonwealth, 1957.
Home Universities Conference, Report of Proceedings, 1952, 1954, 1955, 1956.
Seven Essays on Commonwealth Universities. August 1958.

Bailey, Kenneth C., *History of Trinity College, Dublin.* The University Press, Dublin. 1947.

Baker, J. F., *Engineering Education at Cambridge.* Typewritten copy of address given before Institution of Mechanical Engineers at Cambridge.

Barker, Sir Ernest, *British Universities.* Longmans, Green and Co., Ltd. 1949.

Board of Adult Education, University of Birmingham, *Annual Report of the Director of Extra-Mural Studies, Session 1955–56.* Stanford & Mann, Ltd., Birmingham.

British Council, *Higher Education in the United Kingdom.* Published by the British Council and the Association of Universities of the British Commonwealth. Longmans, Green and Co., rev. ed. 1956.

Cambridge University, Engineering Department, *General Information,* September 1956. Printed in Great Britain at the University Press, Cambridge.

Central Office of Information, Reference Pamphlet 7, *Education in Britain.* Her Majesty's Stationery Office. 1956.

Technological Education in Britain. Pamphlet 21. December 1956. Her Majesty's Stationery Office. 1957.

Coutts, James, *A History of the University of Glasgow.* James Maclehose and Sons, Glasgow. 1909.

Department of Scientific and Industrial Research, *Notes of D.S.I.R. Grants for Graduate Students and Research Workers.* Revised January 1957. Her Majesty's Stationery Office, London.

Donaldson, Alfred Gaston, *Some Comparative Aspects of Irish Law.* Published for the Duke University Commonwealth-Studies Center, Duke University Press, Durham, N. C. 1957.

Dublin, University College, *Report of the President* for the session 1955–56, December 1956. Browne and Nolan, Ltd.

Dudley, D. R., *A Survey of New Developments, 1945–1955.* The Department of Extra-Mural Studies of the University of Birmingham. Stanford & Mann, Ltd., Birmingham.

Education Authority of Glasgow, and others, *Liberal Studies,* a programme of Adult Classes in the City of Glasgow, Session 1956–57. Glasgow Corporation Printing and Stationery Dept.

England, Central Office of Information, *Technological Education in Britain.* Pamphlet prepared by Reference Division, Central Office of Information, London, No. Rf.p.3422. December 1956.

England, Labour, Ministry of, and National Service, *Scientific and Engineering Manpower in Great Britain.* Report of the Office of the Lord President of the Council Ministry of Labour and National Service. H. M. Stationery Office. 1956.

England, Minister of Education, Command Paper #9703, *Technical Education,* February 1956. H. M. Stationery Office, London.

England, Ministry of Education, *Becoming a Teacher.* Curwen Press, London. 1956.

The Educational System of England and Wales. Pamphlet. 1955. (2390/1)

A Career in Education for University Graduates. Pamphlet. 1956. McCorquodale, London.

The Supply and Training of Teachers for Technical Colleges. Report of a special committee appointed by the Minister of Education in September 1956. H. M. Stationery Office. 1957.

Youth's Opportunity, Further Education in County Colleges. Pamphlet No. 3, Her Majesty's Stationery Office. 1946.

Training Colleges in England and Wales Recognized by the Minister. Her Majesty's Stationery Office. 1956.

Evans, D. Emrys, *The University of Wales, Historical Sketch.* Cardiff University of Wales Press. 1953.

Federation of British Industries, *Industry and the Technical Colleges.* Handbook. September 1956. J. W. Arrowsmith, Ltd., Bristol.

Foster, J. F., *Functions of the Association of Universities of the British Commonwealth.* C. F. Hodgson & Son, Ltd. July 1955.

Glasgow, University of, Department of Extra-Mural Education, *Residential Summer School,* Trinity College, Dublin, July 20 to August 3, 1957.
Residential Summer School in Natural Science at St. Mary's College, Durham, July 28 to August 10, 1957.
Annual Report, 1955–56, of Extra-Mural Education Committee. Hedderwick Kirkwood Ltd., Glasgow.
Summer School, Department of Extra-Mural Education, Monday, May 20 to Saturday, May 25, 1957.

Grant, Alexander, *The Story of the University of Edinburgh.* Vols. 1 and 2, London, Longmans, Green and Co. 1884.

Kersting, A. F. and Bryan Little, *Portrait of Cambridge.* B. T. Batsford, Ltd. 1955.

Kneller, G. F., *Higher Learning in Britain.* Cambridge University Press for University Press of California. 1955.

Laurie, S. S., *The Rise of Universities.* Humboldt Library of Science, No. 91. Humboldt Publishing Co., N. Y. May 1887.

Leeds, University of, *Institute of Education Handbook, 1955 and 1956.* William Stevens Limited.
A Decade of Adult Education, 1946–1956. Jowett and Sowry, Ltd., Leeds.
Institute of Education, Researches and Studies, Number 15, January 1957. William Stevens, Ltd.
Institute of Education Annual Report, Session 1955–56; 1948–49; 1949–50; 1950–51; 1954–55.
Institute of Education Bulletins: March 1957; February 1955; March 1954; November 1953; June 1953; March 1953, June 1952.
Department of Adult Education and Extra-Mural Studies, Tenth Annual Report, 1955-56. Jowett & Sowry, Ltd.

Liverpool, University of, Institute of Education, *Prospectus of Courses,* Session 1956-57. C. Tinling & Co., Ltd.

Regulations Affecting Syllabus and Examinations. C. Tinling & Co., Ltd.

Report of the Liverpool University Department of Extra-Mural Studies for the Session 1954–55, November 1955; Session 1953–54, November 1954; and Session 1955-56, November 1956. C. Tinling & Co., Ltd.

Report of the Development Committee to the Council and Senate of the University of Liverpool on Building Progress, 1949–1954. Liverpool University Press. 1955.

Logan, D. W. *The University of London, An Introduction.* The Athlone Press. 1956.

London, University of, *Report by the Principal for the Year 1956–57.* Western Printing Services, Ltd., Bristol.

Longmate, Norman, *Oxford Triumphant.* Phoenix House, Ltd. 1954.

Manchester, University of, *Report of Council to the Court of Governors,* Part 1, November 1956. Morris and Yeaman, Ltd., Manchester.

Ministry of Education, *Education in 1953.* Report of the Ministry of Education and the Statistics of Public Education for England and Wales. Cmd. 9155. H. M. Stationery Office. June 1954.

Education in 1955. Cmd. 9785. July 1956.

Murray, Sir Keith, *The Work of the University Grants Committee in Great Britain.* Reprinted from: "Universiteit en Hogeschool" le Jaargang No. 6, pag. 250–262, 1955.

National Advisory Council on the Training and Supply of Teachers, *Three Year Training for Teachers* (Fifth Report), September 1956. H. M. Stationery Office, London. 1956.

National Foundation for Educational Research in England and Wales, *Tenth Annual Report, 1955–56.* King, Thorne & Stace, Ltd., Brighton.

Statement of Policy, May, 1953.

Bulletin No. 8, November, 1956. King, Thorne & Stace, Ltd., Brighton.

Oliver, R. A. C., *A General Paper in the General Certificate of Education Examination,* July 1954. Occ. Paper #1 (Joint Matriculation Board, Univs. of Manchester, Liverpool, Leeds, Sheffield and Birmingham).

An Experimental Examination in General Studies. December 1955. Morris and Yeaman, Printers, Ltd., Manchester.

Oxford University, Institute of Education, *Handbook, 1955.* The Abbey Press.

Political and Economic Planning Broadsheet No. 357, *Choosing University Students.* P.E.P. 1954.

The Keele Experiment: The University College of North Staffordshire After Four Years. P.E.P. 1954.

Queen's University of Belfast, *Research Students and Higher Degrees and Diploma in Public Health.* Excerpt from Calendar. Pub. by Marjory Boyd, Printer to the Queen's University of Belfast.

Rait, Robert S., *Life in the Medieval University.* Cambridge University Press. 1912.

Ruskin, John, *The Crown of Wild Olive.* Clarke, Given & Hooper, N. Y. n.d.

Scottish Institute of Adult Education, *Scottish Adult Education.* Quarterly. No. 19, April 1957. Walker & Son, Ltd., Printers, Galashiels, University of Edinburgh.

Sinclair, D. C., *Medical Students and Medical Sciences.* Oxford University Press. 1955.

Southern, Richard, *The Dramatic Studio of the University of Bristol.* Pamphlet. n.d.

Tierney, Dr. Michael, *Struggle With Fortune,* Catholic University of Ireland. Browne & Nolan, Ltd. n.d.

Trevelyan, G. M., *History of England.* Volume III, Doubleday & Company, Inc., Garden City, N. Y. 1956.

Truscot, Bruce, *Red Brick University.* Penguin Books. 1951.

Tutorial Classes, Central Joint Advisory Committee, *Forty-Sixth Annual Report,* Session 1954–55. Staples Printers, Ltd., Kent.

Underhill, Frank H., *The British Commonwealth.* Published for the Duke University Commonwealth-Studies Center, Duke University Press, Durham, N. C. 1956.

Universities Council for Adult Education, *Report of the Session 1955–1956.* n.d.

University Grants Committee, *University Development.* Interim

Report on the Years 1952 to 1956. Command Paper #79. H. M. Stationery Office. Cmd. 8875, July 1953, *Univ. Development, Report on the Years 1947 to 1952.*

U.S.A.

Alabama, University of, Alumni News, *American Higher Education, 1958.* Vol. 39, No. 5, March–April 1958.

American Council on Education, *Faculty-Administration Relationships,* Ed. by Frank C. Abbott. Pamphlet. 1958.

International Educational Activities of American Colleges and Universities. Report of the Commission on Education and International Affairs. April 17, 1957. Reprinted from the October 1957 issue of THE EDUCATIONAL RECORD.

Higher Education and National Affairs. Bulletin No. 5, Volume VII. February 5, 1958.

Beatley, Bancroft, *Another Look at Women's Education.* Simmons College, Boston. 1955.

Blegen, Theodore C., *The Harvests of Knowledge.* The Research Foundation of State University of New York, Albany, N. Y. 1957.

Bogue, Jesse P., Ed., *American Junior Colleges,* Fourth Edition, 1956. American Council on Education, Washington 6, D. C. (The George Banta Co., Inc., Menasha, Wisc.)

Bonthius, Robert H., and others, *The Independent Study Program in the United States.* Columbia University Press, N. Y. 1957.

Brown University, *Report to the Corporation of Brown University on Changes in the System of Collegiate Education.* March 28, 1850. Thurston, Torry and Company, Printers, Devonshire Street, Boston.

Carnegie Corporation of New York. *Quarterly Reports:* Vol. V, No. 1, January 1957; Vol. V., No. 2, April 1957; Vol. V, No. 3, July 1957; Vol. VI, No. 1, January 1958; Vol. VI, No. 3, July 1958.

Carnegie Foundation for the Advancement of Teaching. *Annual Reports:* 1946–47; 1948–49; 1949–50; 1950–51; 1951–52; 1952–53; 1953–54.

Circle, The, Vol. 37, No. 3. Spring 1958.

Cole, Fred, *The Impending Tidal Wave of Opportunity.* Address given at the North Carolina College Conference, Winston-Salem N. C., November 7, 1957.

Colville, Derek, *British and American Schools*. Pages 56–62, HARPER'S MAGAZINE, October 1957.

Conant, James B., *Modern Science and Modern Man*. Bampton Lectures in America, No. 5, Delivered at Columbia University, 1952. Columbia University Press, New York. 1952.

Education in the Western World, pages 73–77, THE ATLANTIC MONTHLY, Vol. 200, No. 5, November 1957.

Eddy, Edward Danforth, *Colleges for Our Land and Time*. Harper & Brothers, N. Y. 1957.

Educational Forum, The, Volume XXII, No. 4, May 1958.

Educational Record, The, Volume 39, No. 2, April 1958.

Eurich, Dr. Alvin C., *Opening the Iron Curtains*, BENNINGTON COLLEGE ALUMNAE MAGAZINE, Volume 9, No. 1, 1957.

Ewell, Raymond, *Education and Research in Soviet Russia*. Talk given before the annual meeting of the Textile Research Institute, March 13, 1958.

Flexner, Abraham, *Universities, American, English, German*. Oxford University Press, N. Y. 1930.

Fund for the Advancement of Education, *They Went to College Early*. Evaluation Report No. 2. Pamphlet. April 1957. *A Report for 1954–56*.

Ginn and Company, *What the Colleges are Doing*, No. 111, May 1958.

Iffert, Robert E., *Retention and Withdrawal of College Students*. U. S. Department of Health, Education and Welfare, Bulletin 1958, No. 1. U. S. Govt. Printing Office, Washington. 1957.

Jacob, Philip E., *Changing Values in College*. Harper & Brothers, N. Y. 1957.

Key Reporter, The, Vol. XXIII, No. 1, October 1957.

Klopsteg, Paul E., *University Responsibilities and Government Money*. SCIENCE, Vol. 124, No. 3228, November 9, 1956.

How Shall We Pay for Research and Education? SCIENCE, Vol. 124, No. 3229, November 16, 1956.

Lester, Robert MacDonald, *The Renaissance of Higher Education in the South After 1875*. Pamphlet. 53rd Annual Phi Beta Kappa Address, given before Alpha Chapter of North Carolina, May 14, 1957.

Lovejoy, Clarence E., *Lovejoy's College Guide*. Simon and Schuster, New York. 1956–57.

McKean, Dayton D., *Who's in Charge Here?* Reprinted from THE COLORADO QUARTERLY, Volume VI, Number 4, Spring 1958.

Michigan Council of State College Presidents, *Future School and College Enrollments in Michigan: 1955 to 1970*. J. W. Edwards, Publisher, Inc., Ann Arbor, Michigan. 1954.

Miernyk, William H. and Morris A. Horowitz, *Engineering Enrollment and Faculty Requirements, 1957–67*. (Prepared for the Committee on Development of Engineering Faculties of the American Society for Engineering Education, March 1958.)

Morton, John R., *University Extension in the United States*. University of Alabama Press. 1953.

Nation, The, Volume 186, No. 19, Saturday, May 10, 1958.

National Association of State Universities in the United States of America, *Transactions and Proceedings*, Regular Annual Meeting, The University Club, New York, May 5–6, 1958. Volume LVI, 1958.

National Commission on Accrediting, *Report*. Workshop Conference on Accrediting, June 25–26, 1957. Pamphlet. 1785 Massachusetts Avenue, N.W., Washington 6, D. C.

N.E.A. *Journal*, March, 1958, Vol. 47, No. 3, *The Contemporary Challenge to American Education, Improvement of Teaching*, page 195.

New York, State University of, *Proceedings*, Symposium, January 27–28, 1950, *Functions of a Modern University*. Published by State University of New York, Albany 1, N. Y.

Ortega y Gasset, Jose, *Mission of the University*. Routledge and Kegan Paul. 1946.

Plock, Richard H., *Issues In State Control of Higher Education*. Panel discussion, The Association of Governing Boards of State Universities and Allied Institutions, May 1, 1957.

President's Committee on Education Beyond the High School, *Second Report to the President, July, 1957*. U.S. Govt. Printing Office.

Radio-Electronics, magazine, *The U.S.A. At Bay*, December 1957. *The Elements of Teleducation*, May 1956. *Tec-Teleducation*, February 1955. *Teleducation*, September 1951.

Rockefeller Brothers Fund, Inc., *The Pursuit of Excellence*. Panel Report V, Special Studies Project. Doubleday & Co., Inc., Garden City, New York. 1958.

Rockefeller Foundation, The, *Annual Report, 1956*.

Rockefeller Foundation Grants, Volume VIII, No. 2, Second Quarter, 1957. Pub. by The Rockefeller Foundation, 49 W. 49th St., New York 20, N.Y.

School and Society: V.85, No. 2103, January 19, 1957; V.86, No. 2123, January 4, 1958; V.86, No. 2124, January 18, 1958; V.86, No. 2127, March 1, 1958; V.86, No. 2129, March 29, 1958; V.86, No. 2132, May 10, 1958; V.86, No. 2133, May 24, 1958; V.86, No. 2134, June 7, 1958.

Science, Volume 128, No. 3318, August 1, 1958.

Smith, Seymour A., *Religious Instruction in State Universities*. Reprinted from *Religious Education*, May–June 1958. Religious Education Association, 545 West 111th St., New York 25, N.Y.

Strothmann, F. W., *The Graduate School Today and Tomorrow*. (For Committee of Fifteen.) December 1955. Fund for the Advancement of Education, 477 Madison Ave., N.Y. 22, N.Y.

Tead, Ordway, *The Climate of Learning*. Harper and Brothers, New York. 1958. (John Dewey Society Lecture.)

U.S. Department of Health, Education and Welfare, *Earned Degrees Conferred by Higher Educational Institutions, 1956–57*. Circular No. 527, April 1958.
Engineering Enrollments and Degrees, 1957. Circular No. 516. U.S. Govt. Printing Office, Washington. 1958.
Opening Enrollment in Higher Educational Institutions: Fall, 1957. Circular No. 518, January 1958. U.S. Govt. Printing Office, Washington. 1958.

U.S. Senate Committee on Government Operations, *Science and Technology Act of 1958*. (Committee Print), Analysis and Summary on S.3126. U.S. Govt. Printing Office, Washington. 1958.

Wilson, Louis R., *The University of North Carolina, 1900–30*. University of North Carolina Press. 1957.

Numerous university catalogs and calendars have been consulted in connection with the study.

INDEX

An index of colleges, universities, and institutions follows this topical index.

British universities, *see* Great Britain

Building programs, 294–296 in Australia, 120; in Canada, 114–116; in India, 123; student housing, 133–135; in United Kingdom, 113

Canada, adult education, 271–273; special problems in, 310–311; study of law, 189–191, 311; study of medicine, 195–196; teacher training, 209–210, 217, 223; technical education, 243–246; theological training, 180; universities in, 25–27, 102; women's education, 166, 171–172

Canada Council, 114, 115, 116

Carnegie, Andrew, 16, 47

Carnegie Foundation, 200, 275–276

Chief executive officers, influence of, 98–100; titles of, 97–99

Church influence, in founding universities, 107, 117; in teacher training, 205, 206, 207

Church sponsorship of higher education, 2, 27

Church work, *see* Theology, practical

Ctizenship, as goal of education, 83

Civic universities in Britain, 18–24, 64, 68, 89–90

Civil Code, 190, 311

Civil Law, 190, 191, 311

Clergy, training of, *see* Theology

Clubs, departmental, 144–145, 155–156

Coeducation, earliest, xviii; in U.S. state universities, 165, 304–306

Colleges, community, 57–58, 315; defined in U.S., 47; junior, 39, 40, 42, 56–58, 66–67, 315; for women, 158, 160, 162, 163, 164,

165, 166, 170, 171, 172; *see also* University

Commission on University Education, proposal for, 340–341

Common Law, 190, 191, 311

Commonwealth countries, difference from U.S. education aim, 74; honors degrees in, 70–73, 67; women's colleges in, 157–161, 166, 170, 185

Commonwealth universities, growth of, 37–38

Communication, need for between professions, 334

Community colleges, *see* Colleges, community

Community service, 280–282; *see also* Adult education *and* Research

Compensation of teachers, 218, 297–298

Compulsory education of girls, 160, 161

Conant, President James B., 80, 328

Controls, government, on higher education, 320–324

Counseling, student, 132, 139–142, 153–154

Court of Governors, 86, 88, 89

Criticism, of modern British university, 74–75, 300, 304–305, 308–310

Curricula, changes in U.S., 51–52; engineering, 253–254; growth of, 63–66; as heritage of Western culture, 326–329; in land-grant colleges, 49–50; in study of law, 188–192; in study of medicine in India, 198–200, 203; technical, 231, 233, 237–247, 253, 256–258; for study of theology, 178, 179, 182, 184, 185; in U.S. arts colleges, 39–40; for women, 304–306; in Commonwealth countries, 167–

Funds, available for U.S. medical schools, 201–202; refused by Quebec universities, 115, 311, 323

General education, *see* Education, general
Gifted students, 3, 221, 293, 301–304
Girls, *see* Women
Goal of university education, 84, 173–174, 257, 300
Goals of arts faculties, 324–326
Government, student, 144, 145, 146
Government grants, Commonwealth compared to U.S., 125–126; earmarked for science, 322; for higher education, *see* University income
Government support of education, 21, 111–129, 319–320, 321–323; in Australia, 118–120; effect on autonomy, 4, 127–130; in South Africa, 120–122; *see also* University Grants Commission *and* University Grants Committee
Great Britain, adult education, 259–271; curricula in universities, 64–65, 68; educational experiments in, 75–76; elementary education, 204–205; medical and health facilities, 137–138; special problems in, 308–310; sports in universities, 136; study of law in, 185, 187–189, 191; study of medicine in, 194–195, 203; teacher training in, 204–209, 222; technical education in, 225–239; theological training in, 178–180; university income, 112–114, 127; women's education, 157–161, 166, 167, 169, 172–173, 185
Great Issues Course, 155

Griswold, A. Whitney, quoted, 73
Guidance, student, 97, 132, 139–142, 153–154
Guidance program, improvements needed, 337

Harper, President Rainey, 41, 56–57
Health, student, 132, 137–139
Heritage, reflected in curriculum, 326–329
Higher education, *see* Education
Higher education for women, *see* Women
Higher Learning in Britain, 60–61
Hindi as language of instruction, 313–314
Home, as basic to education, 176
Homemaking, preparation for, 78, 162, 163, 167, 168, 169, 170, 171, 172, 174, 175, 176
Honor societies, 146–147
Honors courses, gifted student and, 293
Honors degrees, in Commonwealth countries, 70–73, 76; in Great Britain, 16, 82, 308
Housing, student, 131, 133–135, 294–296
Housing for women, 304, 306
Human relations, as world problem, 175–176
Humanities, as adult education, 261, 266, 267, 269–270, 271–274; emphasized at Oxford, 14; need for, 332, 333, 335; at New South Wales University of Technology, 28–29; place in modern curricula, 327–329; required study of, 68–69; by engineering students, 244, 246, 249, 256–258; by medical students, 195, 196–197; studied by foreign exchange students, 153; studied in Russia, 305; at technological in-

Colleges, Universities and Institutions

Set in Linotype Caledonia
Format by James T. Parker
Manufactured by The Riverside Press
Published by HARPER & BROTHERS, *New York*